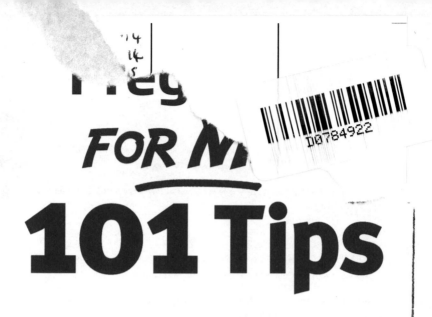

Preg...
FOR ME...

101 Tips

Mark Woods

white
LADDER

H46 532 860 9

Pregnancy for Men: 101 Tips

This first edition published in 2012 by White Ladder, an imprint of Crimson Publishing Ltd, Westminster House, Kew Road, Richmond, Surrey, TW9 2ND

Content in this book has been previously published in *Pregnancy for Men* © Mark Woods, 2010

© Mark Woods, 2012

The right of Mark Woods to be identified as the author of this work has been asserted by him in accordance with the Copyright, Designs and Patents Act, 1988.

All rights reserved. This book is sold subject to the condition that it shall not, by way of trade or otherwise, be lent, resold, hired out or otherwise circulated without the publisher's prior written consent in any form of binding or cover other than that in which it is published and without a similar condition including this condition being imposed on the subsequent purchaser. No part of this publication may be reproduced, stored in a retrieval system or transmitted in any form or by any means, electronic and mechanical, photocopying, recording or otherwise without prior permission of Crimson Publishing.

British Library Cataloguing in Publication Data

A catalogue record for this book is available from the British Library.

ISBN 978 1 90828 130 2

Typeset by IDSUK (DataConnection) Ltd
Printed and bound in the UK by TJ International Ltd, Padstow, Cornwall

To Sarah and the boys, 101 kisses.

Introduction

At last count there were around 230 million books (or something like that) written to help pregnant women through what is, by anyone's standards, a remarkable nine months as they carry their first baby.

The times they are a-changing though and while as recently as the late 1960s and early 1970s the father of the soon-to-be arriving child was all but barred from the delivery room, we now live in a world where upwards of 90% of UK births happen with the male partner present.

That's a very big shift.

Of course it's not just the labour ward where men are becoming more active – an ever-increasing number of us want to be involved, want to play our part, and want to really help during pregnancy and beyond.

I wrote *Pregnancy for Men* in an attempt to redress this bedside-table book imbalance that many fathers-to-be notice – and it seems to have been worth doing.

But in a world where we are increasingly bombarded with more information than we could ever possibly know what to do with, the version you are holding in your hands aims to boil things down to the brass tacks.

Taking the 101 most pertinent pieces of wisdom from *Pregnancy for Men* – all of which have been gleaned from our fellow fathers and an ocean of research and studies – this book is designed for the man who has so little time, reading anything longer than a 140-character tweet represents a colossal undertaking.

So, flick, dip, do the lot at once and go back when the time comes – however you read them, I hope these tips help you and your partner enjoy pregnancy and prepare you for the extraordinary and never-to-be-forgotten moment when you will be transformed from being a mere man, to being somebody's dad.

Month 1

1

Don't panic

The NHS estimates that of 100 couples trying to conceive naturally:

- 20 will conceive within one month

- 70 will conceive within six months

- 85 will conceive within one year

- 90 will conceive within 18 months

- 95 will conceive within two years.

(If, by the way, you've added up the numbers on the left and are trying to fathom out why they come to 360 rather than 100, you should perhaps be asking yourself whether children are really a wise move.)

2

Avoid the lube boob

Many of the more popular brands of personal lubricant seriously inhibit the ability of sperm to get where it needs to go.

There are some special sexual lubricants on the market which claim to have overcome this problem, as it were, so it's definitely worth a bit of research if you lube up when trying for a baby.

3

Test me, test me

Make no mistake: your reaction to the positive pregnancy test result will be remembered, regurgitated and requoted for decades to come.

For the love of God, don't let any fear or anxiety you may be feeling turn into words at that precise moment. If you're feeling like the contents of your stomach have divided equally and are heading to both your north and south orifices, keep it to yourself and tell her later after the initial moment has passed.

It's an overwhelming thing to find out that you are on your way to being a dad and it has the potential to mess with your head for a second or two, but be positive and warm, she's probably twice as scared as you are and the last thing she needs is you screaming 'Shiiiiiit'. Besides there's plenty of time to worry yourself sick later – just enjoy this moment.

4

Keeping mum, mum

The three-month silence that many couples take part in about their pregnancy news is a far from universal or uniform practice.

Many people choose to tell parents or close friends, as much to gain early support in the tough first few weeks as the desire to spread the joy.

There is no right or wrong way of doing it, just what suits you and the mother of your child best.

5

The M word

The often-quoted figure is that around 20% of all pregnancies end in miscarriage, but this is increasingly being seen as a woefully conservative estimation.

Many miscarriages can and do happen without women even realising they were pregnant, putting the episode down to a heavier than usual period.

With that taken into account, the miscarriage rate is thought to be more like 40% or 50% – with some experts going as far as to say that almost every sexually active woman will have one at some point in her life, whether she is aware of it or not.

Whatever the true figure is, what's for sure is that miscarriage lurks around the first three months of pregnancy like a menacing playground bully; probably never likely to strike, but always a threat.

6

Morning, afternoon and evening sickness

Nausea and sickness can and do strike a pregnant woman at any time of the day, or even at night.

It's reckoned around eight out of 10 mothers-to-be feel sick at some point, with half of them actually vomiting. Symptoms vary wildly from woman to woman. The lucky ones will get the odd bout of mild queasiness, whereas others will be struck down by the severest, truly debilitating form of the complaint.

If your partner suffers from this, you are both in for a tough time. She will be vomiting morning, noon and night, unable to eat and drink properly, and even losing weight when she should be putting it on.

7

Steadying the ship

If your partner does suffer from morning sickness there are things you can do to help.

- Encourage your partner to avoid drinks that are cold, tart or sweet and to drink little and often, rather than in large amounts.

- If she eats small, frequent meals that are high in carbohydrate and low in fat she could avoid the worse bouts.

- Apparently if she eats some plain dry biscuits 20 minutes before she gets out of bed, it works wonders! This tip seems to get passed on from generation to generation and is, if nothing else, a good excuse to snack in bed.

- Avoid piping-hot meals – clever one, this. Cold food doesn't give off as much of a smell as hot food.

8

What a month!

At the end of its first month your baby will be about the size of a raisin; but what a raisin!

Once the fertilised egg is embedded in the lining of the uterus, it multiplies and grows at an astonishing rate. What was originally a sperm/egg combo is now officially a blastocyst (fluid-filled ball) comprising several hundred cells.

Pretty soon though this blastocyst divides into two.

The half still attached to the womb will become the placenta – unlucky. The other half will become your baby – jackpot.

Month 2

9

Help take the strain

Women who suffer from chronic constipation during pregnancy are often truly plagued. Irregular bowel movements and sluggish, turgid intestines can make their lives, well, shit really. And when constipation's sidekick from hell – haemorrhoids – pops up, or out as the case may be, then things really do turn nasty.

Here are three key ways you can help your partner avoid a major logjam though.

- Fibre is your best mate in the fight against constipation. Plenty of fresh fruit and vegetables, wholegrain cereals and breads, legumes and dried fruit, all help to get things moving. But, for the sake of the neighbours, don't let her jump right in to a fibre-rich diet if it's a departure from the norm – she will develop wind and bloating like you would not believe.

- Eating six mini-meals a day rather than three full-blown ones can make a significant difference.

- Water, fruit and vegetable juices not only get things moving, but soften the stool so when it does finally make an appearance it's not like passing a pine cone.

10

And relax

Pregnant women get very, very, very tired and the best way to cope with this tiredness is simple.

Give in.

That sounds straightforward, but of course it isn't. If your partner loves her job or can't bear to miss out on what her friends are up to, she may well fight it for a while, but both work and social engagements eventually have to come second to the relentless waves of exhaustion that early pregnancy can bring.

You can help here in a big way by encouraging a reduction of her list of daily activities right down to the essentials, stocking the fridge with healthy ready meals, turning down the odd social do and making it possible for her to fit in a daily nap.

It's also worth bearing in mind that once the baby is born you will be begging on hands and knees for just four hours of continuous sleep – so the pair of you should make hay and kip like nobody's business while you still can.

11

Keep smiling

As we've seen, it's fair to say that pregnancy brings with it an eruption of hormonal activity on a volcanic scale. Almost every symptom, every change, is driven by a heady cocktail of chemicals – the word hormone itself means 'to spur on' and you can see why.

This potent pregnancy piñacolada unsurprisingly also leads to mood swings and heightened emotions of all types for the mother-to-be. Of course this is all played out against a backdrop of the whole gambit of feelings that having a baby throws up too – joy, fear, worry, excitement – they are all there in spades, so pour on a canful of petrol of hectic hormones too and it's little wonder that the odd tear is shed.

And that's just by you.

Then of course there are arguments. Even though it's really, really hard at times to avoid a row with someone who is crying at the weather forecast one minute and screaming at a cupboard that refuses to open smoothly the next, the onus is on you to take one for the team, swallow the bitter pill of righteousness and end any rifts quickly.

Think of the children, man, think of the children.

12

Sex. There, I said it

With a normal pregnancy, having sex is safe right until your partner's waters break. Unless you have a traffic cone for a penis there is no way you can hit, prod, nudge or poke your baby.

Surrounded by amniotic fluid, shielded by a drawbridge-like cervix and sealed by a mucus plug, your offspring is incredibly well protected and an ample but limited appendage like the one we all carry around with us just doesn't have what it takes to gatecrash the pregnancy party.

There are, though, certain circumstances that can make sex during pregnancy unsafe. Women who have any of these health complications should seek medical advice before doing the do:

- a previous premature birth

- leaking amniotic fluid

- a history or high risk of miscarriage

- unexplained vaginal bleeding, discharge or cramping

- placenta praevia (a condition in which the placenta is low and covers the cervix)

- incompetent cervix (when the cervix is weakened and opens too soon).

13

Tuck her in

Changing bed linen is a job with a very high pain-in-the-arse rating – every man knows that.

Every man also knows just how much better you sleep on lovely, cool, new sheets though.

Chances are your partner is more exhausted right now than she has ever been in her life.

You know what to do.

14

The cat's done a whoopsy

Cat crap can pose a very real danger to your pregnant partner. A horrid shit-inhabiting bug called Toxoplasma gondii lurks in cat faeces, as well as in unwashed fruit and veg.

If caught by a pregnant woman it can be transferred from her via the placenta to her baby. The infection has the potential to cause miscarriage, blindness in the foetus or damage to its nervous system.

If you've got a cat, emptying the litter tray is your job now my old son.

15

The incredible expanding baby

By the end of this second month, your baby will be four times the size it was at the start of it. That is quite a growth spurt, by anyone's standards. Having said that, even after expanding at such an indecent rate, the little fella is still about the length of a fun-sized Mars bar.

All major organs develop in this intense period and the heart, although no bigger than a peppercorn, begins to beat strongly. Wrists and fingers begin to appear on the end of the still-forming arms, and legs start to develop with, amazingly, tiny little toes already appearing on the ends.

Under the baby's paper-thin skin its face starts to take shape too; bones fuse, the beginnings of a nose is formed and the outlines of the cheeks and a jaw can be seen. Inside his mouth sits a minute tongue.

Genitals have even begun to develop.

All this on a mini Mars bar.

Month 3

16

Become a scan fan

Ultrasound scans have been used in pregnancy for around 30 years now and have an exemplary safety record, with no side effects being found whatsoever. They work by sending high-frequency sound waves through the womb, which bounce off your baby before being turned into an image on a screen.

Hard tissues such as bone reflect the biggest echoes and show up white, with soft tissues coming out grey. Fluids, such as the amniotic fluid that your baby lies in, come up black as the waves pass right through them.

Sonographers (scanner operators) interpret these images, or failing that, guess. Apart from the gel being a little chilly on her tummy, the only real discomfort caused to your partner is down to the curious fact that to obtain a better picture she needs to have a full bladder while it takes place.

17

It's a date

All pregnant women should be offered a dating scan when they are between 10 and 14 weeks pregnant. As the name suggests, this is primarily to nail down exactly how pregnant your partner is in a bid to avoid her going full term in Sainsbury's when she actually thinks she still has a month to go.

Also, because hormones vary at different stages of pregnancy, pinning down exactly what stage she is at is vital for future tests to be valid.

That isn't all the scan does though; it can check that your baby has a regular heartbeat and is developing normally – which is always nice to know, isn't it? Your baby's head, hands, feet and limbs can all be seen after a fashion and even some organs can be viewed.

18

How many!

Out of 781,000 births in the UK in 2009, 12,595 were twins, with 172 triplets and five sets of quadruplets being born.

Keep your eyes on that scan screen!

19

The light of my wife

There's going to be a lot of late-night weeing going on in your house from now on with are expectant mother having her bladder put under increasing pressure from the growing baby in her tummy.

Putting a small light in the path of your partner's route to the loo so she can see where she is going is a sensible move.

Sweeping the route before you go to bed for any dangerous items she might trip over is smart too.

20

Take her away from it all

The beginning of this third month can be a brute for your partner; little or no let-up in symptoms, scans on the horizon and six more months to go – yeesh!

Booking a night away in a quiet hotel will go down a treat, or if money is tight, a candlelit night in with you waiting on her hand and foot before making time to talk about any worries she might have, will be long remembered.

21

Class act

This one is a blinder.

Antenatal classes might seem a long way off in the seventh month or so, but the best ones get booked up way ahead of time. The sessions run by the National Childbirth Trust (NCT) get snapped up especially quickly and have – rightly or wrongly – more of a reputation for forging long-lasting friendships among parents than some of the NHS-run ones.

Get online, get on the phone, find out the details and watch the mother-to-be of your child melt in admiration as you tell her you've been doing a bit of research into parenting classes.

22

Perfect miniature

By the end of this third month your baby is fully formed. Job done, the show's over, move along, nothing more to see here.

Well not quite – there's still a large amount of growth needed.

But all of your baby's major organs have formed and his intestines have even been packed away neatly in his abdomen. He has nails on his toes and fingers and could even have some hair.

The little champ has even started drinking. Not being able to get out much, it's more of a quiet one at home swallowing amniotic fluid and weeing it out like a good 'un.

23

Your little gymnast

There's some serious movement going on at this stage – knee jerks, back twists and the odd all-body hiccup – not that your partner will be able to feel any of that yet. Oh, and your baby can also smile, frown and suck his thumb if he is so inclined.

All this awesome development means that from now on your baby will be at less risk because the critical phase of growth has passed.

You can breathe a little easier from now on.

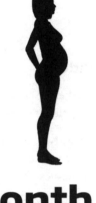

Month 4

24

Beware bottom feeders

Oily fish is good for both mother-to-be and the developing baby, but there is a risk of high levels of pollutants, especially mercury.

It's best to have no more than two portions a week of the likes of mackerel, trout and sardines, so all the benefits are reaped without chancing overexposure to any nasties.

The old cupboard staple of tuna should be limited to no more than four medium-size cans or two tuna steaks a week. Swordfish, marlin and shark should be off the menu altogether – both eating them and swimming with them.

25

Say goodbrie

Blue cheese or types that are soft mould-ripened, such as Brie or Camembert, are to be avoided.

Unpasteurised soft cheeses, such as those made from sheep's or goat's milk should also be consigned to your partner's 'The first thing I'm going to have when it's out' list, if she's a fan.

26

Well done

Eating meat is fine, but make sure it's well cooked with no pink or red bits.

Should Britain ever have a summer to speak of again, take special care when eating barbecued food. Cured meat products, such as salami, are also best avoided.

27

Booze

Mmmm, alcohol and pregnancy. The advice on this seems to change on a daily basis but what's for sure is that no one really knows what a safe level of alcohol consumption is for a pregnant woman.

The most comprehensively safe course of action is for your partner to go on the wagon either for the whole thing or for the first three months when your baby is doing most of its developing.

If giving up booze completely for the entire duration is just too much to bear for her, then the advice is to stick at no more than one or two units of alcohol, no more than once or twice a week.

28

Exercising for two

Exercising is still important for the pregnant woman, even when anatomically it looks like the last thing they should be doing. Care is needed though and if you can help your partner to remember the following, she won't go far wrong.

- Exercise doesn't have to be strenuous to be beneficial – that walk to the shops counts too. As long as it's not the chip shop.

- She should drink plenty of fluids when exercising.

- It's also wise to take a gentle approach to exercise that doesn't put strain on her joints and ligaments.

- Exercising during pregnancy isn't about losing weight.

- She shouldn't exercise flat on her back, particularly after 16 weeks, because her bump presses on the big blood vessels, which isn't a good idea at all.

- Don't use saunas or steam rooms, they make you too hot, and could poach your baby.

29

Fly baby

Flying in the first and second trimesters is generally safe for pregnant women.

The third trimester is out though because not even the most accommodating of flight attendants wants to deliver a baby using a plastic spoon and the whistle from a lifejacket.

Be warned too, ticket agents don't tend to ask if you're pregnant when you book your seats, the little blighters, but there's every chance your partner could be questioned about her due date as she waddles up to the gate – and airlines are well within their rights to bar you from travel if they think there's a chance your partner might ruin the upholstery.

To confirm it's safe for you to fly it's smart to get written permission from your doctor if you can. If the pregnancy is complicated by medical problems you would do well to check with your GP before travelling at any stage.

30

What's the colour of mummy?

Hair colour! Yes hair colour. It might not seem like a big deal to you, but what seems like thousands of online message boards hum with the white-hot chat of whether dying your hair is bad for your baby.

Annoyingly, no one has enough information to say with absolute cast-iron certainty that using a lovely rusty red or mahogany brown during pregnancy is completely and utterly safe.

Animal studies have been carried out over the years, and some, but by no means all, have shown a handful of the chemical compounds in hair dyes do cause birth defects. In most cases though the animals were given doses way, way beyond what women would be exposed to.

With all this unsatisfactory information about, there's no wonder this issue always turns up like a bad penny – but the consensus at the moment is that if the dyes are applied safely, using gloves in a well-ventilated room, and not leaving solutions on for any great length of time, it probably is safe.

31

Tearing a strip off

As hair growth tends to increase for some women during pregnancy, this is another one that comes up more than you'd imagine.

There's no evidence to show that waxing is unsafe during pregnancy and if, like I did, you are wondering if the baby feels an agonising shock as the strips are removed – apparently they don't, so rest easy.

Your partner on the other hand could well be in for a rougher ride than usual because her skin may become even more sensitive in pregnancy.

32

Brush strokes

Is painting during pregnancy safe?

No one really knows.

There's no doubt that painting does expose you to some pretty hefty chemicals, but because it's next to impossible to measure how much the body absorbs, calculating the risks is equally as tricky.

There is some evidence though that exposure to the type of chemical solvents found in paint does increase the chances of birth defects.

There are guidelines for those women who do choose to paint, such as limiting the amount of time you spend doing it, keeping the windows open and wearing long garments to protect the skin; but by far the simplest and safest answer is for your partner to let someone else do the painting.

That means you by the way.

33

Me too

Phantom pregnancy, or couvade syndrome, as this phenomenon has been coined (it's from the French word meaning 'to hatch'), has been documented throughout the ages and some studies put the number of expectant dads who suffer from it in some shape or form as high as 65%.

The condition presents itself in men with symptoms such as nausea, vomiting, stomach pain, back pain, toothache and exhaustion. For many the symptoms are pretty subtle; a spot of weight gain here, an unexplained ache or pain there.

Other men though have full-blown mirror pregnancies, having exactly the same symptoms at exactly the same time as their wives.

34

Hormonal, moi?

A Canadian study found that testosterone levels dropped by a third in new dads during the first three weeks after the baby arrived.

So, essentially mother nature has found a way to engineer it so that the chemical that makes you such a chest-beating, arse-pinching fool of a man, reduces dramatically just at the very time that you need to bond and coo over your newborn baby.

35

What did you just say?

Be warned, your baby can now hear you.

Fair enough, it might not be able to make any sense out of which profanity you just launched towards the wobbly cyclist at the traffic lights, but thanks to its hardening inner ear bones, your little one has begun to pick up its first sounds – which at this stage are mainly your partner's soothing heartbeat, rumbling digestion and all-important voice.

36

All heart

Despite still being only around 14cm in length and weighing in at not much more than 7oz by the end of this fourth month your tiny mite has already developed some pretty impressive skills.

For a start, lung development is steaming ahead and your baby is essentially doing breathing exercises, ready for the big moment when he will take his first breath once the umbilical cord has been cut. As these exercises happen your little one's chest rises and falls as his lungs begin to exhale amniotic fluid.

Not to be left behind, the tiny heart is now capable of pumping an astonishing 24 litres of blood a day too.

37

We feel you baby

There's a good chance that towards the end of this month your partner (but not you yet) will be able to feel the baby moving for the first time.

It's not the thumping great kicks that will boot you out of the bed in months to come, but a fluttering sensation that's been likened to having a swarm of butterflies flying around in your stomach.

Or alternatively, wind.

38

Me Tarzan

During the second and third trimesters the slightest fall for your partner can lead to some pretty serious problems.

It sounds obvious, but gently suggest that you are now the chief lifter and mover in the household.

39

Dear diary

As the baby starts to move it's not a bad idea for your partner to keep a rough record of what she feels when.

Buying her a journal that she can use to do just that is a good move and once baby is born she can use it to keep a track of feeds, sleeps, poos and, crucially, who has done the early shift most times each week.

40

Mummy yoga

Pregnancy yoga is fast becoming a very popular part of the pregnancy routine for many mums-to-be – and with good reason.

As well as being a gentle way to relax as her body goes through a myriad of changes, it's also a great way for your partner to meet other women who are going through the same thing.

Get yourself online and research a few courses in your area – she'll love you for it.

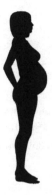

Month 5

41

Top to toe

The 20-week 'anomaly scan' takes less than half an hour to perform but in that time checks your baby's heart, head, spine and kidneys as well as the position of the placenta and the amount of amniotic fluid they have to move around in.

That's a serious MOT.

42

Turtle or hamburger?

The 20-week scan is often when you can choose to find out the sex of your baby too and an experienced sonographer will be on the lookout for one of two signs if you ask them to tell you.

In a girl the three lines that make up the clitoris surrounded by the labia are often charmingly referred to as the hamburger sign. In a boy it's the turtle sign they are watching out for, where the tip of the penis just peeks out from the testicles.

It could just as well have been called the walnut whip.

43

The babymoon

Taking a middle-trimester holiday has become very popular – with your partner neither feeling too sick nor too enormous it's the best time to have your last child-free vacation for a long while.

When choosing your destination though it's worth remembering that many vaccines are off limits and in the case of areas with a high risk of malaria, pregnant women need to think very hard before they travel, as they are especially vulnerable to the killer disease.

Pregnancy makes women more susceptible to malaria infection and increases the risk of illness, severe anaemia and even death. For the unborn child, maternal malaria increases the risk of miscarriage, stillbirth, premature delivery and low birth weight.

It's not to be messed with.

44

Constant craving

Cravings really happen.

A recent survey asked more than 2,000 women if they craved a certain foodstuff or taste while they were expecting and more than 75% said they had.

Half a century ago the figure was at about 30%. So what's going on?

In short, despite a few whacky theories, no one really has a clue.

45

More tea, darling?

There's no easy way to tell you this, but your partner will almost certainly pass more wind from both ends during her pregnancy than you hitherto dreamed possible.

The reason for this often sudden increase in gas, as our American brethren are wont to call it, isn't because she can no longer be bothered to pretend she's saintly in that direction, it's actually down to two separate little wind-generating factors.

Firstly, the hormone progesterone slows down digestion and generates bloating and lots and lots of wind. Secondly, round about month 5, as the baby slowly starts to crowd your partner's insides, her digestive system takes another pounding as it gets squeezed leading to an even higher food-to-flatulence ratio.

46

Baby brain

Over the past decade a number of studies have begun to suggest that baby brain, or mumnesia as it's also been called, is a nailed-on pregnancy symptom, allowing scores of women to relax about the fact that after putting the car keys in the washing machine they struggled for a full 15 minutes to remember their own husband's name to ask if he'd seen them.

Others angrily suggest that the very notion is as patronising and sexist an assertion as is possible.

You decide.

47

Brain box

After weeks of relentless growth, once your baby reaches the five-month stage and is roughly 19cm long, the rate of expansion reduces somewhat (although his weight gain doesn't) and he focusses on other crucial areas of his development – like growing brain cells.

At the centre of his new little brain an area called the germinal matrix is busy manufacturing cells at an almighty rate. The production line stops before birth, but your baby's brain will keep on expanding until around the age of five years.

And then they will go to school.

48

Curd and turd

A thick white greasy substance, not unlike cottage cheese, is starting to cover your baby's body right about now.

Don't fret though – called vernix, this wonderful substance acts as a waterproof barrier to prevent his skin from becoming waterlogged in the sea of amniotic fluid he finds himself floating in.

If only he had a stick of celery or carrot baton in there he could have himself his first ever snack too.

Meanwhile a little welcome gift of baby's first ever turd is also progressing beautifully, as a delightful tar-like substance called meconium accumulates in his bowels.

The shape of things to come.

49

Magic hands

A spot of smart forward planning.

In the coming weeks, various parts of your partner's body are going to ache, creak, lumber and throb like never before as the strain of carrying round a small person in her abdomen starts to really crank up. Be warned, you will be called upon, on a regular basis, to massage said body.

If, like most of us, your idea of a massage is 15 seconds of Chinese burn followed by a few karate chops, it might be a good idea to either do some internet research on a few gentle but effective massage techniques or sign yourself up to a quick course to learn the basics.

50

Eau my god

The vast majority of us are dehydrated according to research. Drinking enough water is something almost everyone in almost every developed country is spectacularly piss-poor at.

While this is bad news for us all, as a pregnant woman it's to be addressed straightaway as water helps to carry nutrients to the baby and also helps to prevent infections, constipation and the dreaded piles.

To help your partner drink the three pints of fluid she needs (coffee, tea and pop don't count I'm afraid as they make you wee more out than they put in), make up jugs of water with wedges of lemon or lime in to help her overcome water boredom. If she hits you with the old 'But I'm suffering from water retention' line, sweetly remind her that the more water she drinks, the less her body will retain.

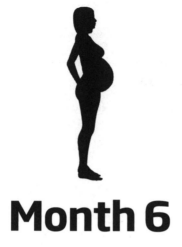

Month 6

51

Six months means . . .

There's more of the pregnancy behind you at this stage than there is still to come.

DON'T PANIC THOUGH!

52

Does my bump look big in this?

If you are glancing nervously at your partner as you read this thinking, 'She hasn't got much of a bump', for Christ's sake keep that thought in your head and out of your big mouth.

The shape, size and position of each bump is as unique as the baby inside it, but that doesn't stop some pretty fierce comparisons taking place between mums-to-be, or even with the odd non-pregger total stranger pitching in to give their tummy two pence as well.

In terms of advice about the size and shape of the bump, the only person who is worth listening to about this outward sign of the inward baby is your partner's midwife.

53

Making a move

From the sixth month onwards many women start to feel the baby hiccupping as it necks pint after pint of its favourite amniotic brew. As the weeks roll on the frequency and type of movements increase dramatically, as does the basic brute force with which they are delivered.

In the later weeks of pregnancy many a man has been awoken from his slumber by a boot or a jab from within the womb. Waking up startled to realise that your unborn child has just landed one on you is one of life's more surreal experiences.

In the final few weeks the baby assumes the position, hopefully head down, limiting himself to the odd punch and kick to the ribs as he waits upside down for disembarkation.

54

This is your father speaking

There was a time, not all that long ago, when leaning into your partner's tummy and talking to your unborn baby was seen as being right up there on the pottiness scale with Prince Charles debating with his dahlias.

Now though, scientists are pretty convinced that at around this stage of the pregnancy the baby is capable of learning to recognise the voice of not only his mother-to-be, but his father-to-be too, as well as pieces of oft-repeated music.

So get chatting to your child right now; it's never too early to start the indoctrination process toward your football club.

55

Contraction comedian

You'd imagine the last thing a women needs as she approaches the great unknown of labour for the very first time is her body sending her a few pretend contractions just to keep her on her toes. But that's pretty much what happens in the shape of Braxton Hicks contractions, named after John Braxton Hicks, an English doctor who first discovered this most cruel of all practical jokes in the late 19th century.

Towards the middle of the pregnancy, or sometimes even earlier, your partner may well start to notice the muscles of her uterus tightening for up to a minute or two.

Usually painless, they can cause the abdomen to become hard and even contorted, and as the delivery date draws closer they helpfully become more frequent, more intense and more like real contractions, just to really get your partner going. Some women don't get them at all; some poor souls can have them come on several times an hour.

56

Money and lots of it

Are you sitting down? Good. Here are a few financial home truths for you.

According to various pieces of research, parents in Britain spend an average of £13,696 in their baby's first year, once childcare and loss of earnings are taken into account.

Even with many mums going back to work after 12 months or so, the average baby spend for the second year weighs in at £4,305, and £4,998 for the third year.

In fact the average cost of raising a child from birth to the age of 21 has been calculated to be more than £210,000. That's £833 a month. Every month. For 21 years.

57

Buying a buggy

Before you enter the stroller solar system and attempt to buy yourself a pram/pushchair combo here's a few tips.

- Ask your friends who have already been there and get their advice.

- Newborn babies need to lie back straight, as their malleable spines can be damaged if they are kept curved for any great length of time, so take that into account.

- Think about where your baby is going to sleep, as this may affect what you buy.

- If you live in a flat, have a normal-sized car, get the bus or train every now and then, or don't happen to have biceps the size of Anglesey, then seriously, seriously think about the size and weight of what you buy. Your back is going to be well and truly buggered as it is carrying a baby around for six months without having to fold and unfold an armoured personnel carrier five times a day too.

58

Very important papa

In recent years study after study has shown that how we perform as fathers profoundly affects how our boys and girls turn into men and women.

- Very young children who spend more time playing with their dads are often more sociable when they enter nursery school.

- Involvement of dads with children aged 7–11 predicts success in exams at 16.

- Where dads are involved before the age of 11, children are less likely to have a criminal record by the age of 21.

- It's even been found that babies who miss out on regular baths by their fathers are more likely to grow up with social problems!

No pressure then.

59

The thinking man's baby

Congratulations, your baby is now capable of conscious thought and can both learn and remember.

Whether he or she can hold a grudge at this point remains unclear though.

60

Give her a wedgie

Stick 'pregnancy wedge pillow' into Google, and if your partner hasn't already got one, get her one.

She gets to support her bump in bed, and yet again you look like the best father-to-be a gal could ever wish for.

61

At a stretch

Stretch marks affect between 75% and 90% of pregnant women. The combination of more weight and higher levels of hormones making the skin thinner than usual is a pain, and can cause some serious anguish and anxiety for many women both during and after pregnancy.

Tips to help keep the skin healthy and supple abound: rubbing the skin with olive oil, vitamin E-rich cream or royal jelly, and drinking lots of water.

There's a good chance though that despite your loving and magic fingers your partner may well develop a permanent stretch mark or two. Your role then is simple; tell her you love her and that she is beautiful, every single day.

62

Floor it

In motivational terms, the reasons for your partner doing pelvic floor exercises are about as compelling as they come. They help:

- protect her from incontinence during and after pregnancy

- support the extra weight of pregnancy and may even help shorten the second stage of labour

- heal the perineum after birth

- achieve orgasm during sex.

Makes you wonder why we aren't all doing them en masse in the work car park every morning, doesn't it?

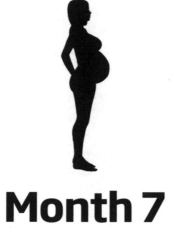

Month 7

63

Mantenatal

If you are undecided about going to antenatal classes here's my advice.

Go.

You might feel bored, you might feel uncomfortable, you might have to pretend to be friends with lots of people.

But you'll almost certainly learn at least one piece of information you'll use during the labour – which has to make it a must.

64

Home births

In 1955, there were 683,640 births in England and Wales, of which 33.4% took place at home.

In 2010, of the 679,638 babies born, a mere 2.5% arrived at home, the vast majority born in hospitals and other medical institutions.

If you and your partner favour a home birth the chances are you are going to have to fight for one and hold your nerve.

65

Zzzzzzzzz

Prolonged sleep deprivation has been used as a means of interrogation, most famously by the KGB.

Menachem Begin, the Prime Minister of Israel from 1977 to 1983, who was unfortunate enough to have experienced the technique while a prisoner in Russia, described it as follows:

'In the head of the interrogated prisoner, a haze begins to form. His spirit is wearied to death, his legs are unsteady, and he has one sole desire: to sleep . . . Anyone who has experienced this desire knows that not even hunger and thirst are comparable with it.'

SLEEP NOW, WHILE YOU STILL CAN.

66

Premature births aren't as rare as you think

More than 50,000 babies are born prematurely each year in the UK, which equates to around one in eight deliveries.

Pre-term is defined as being born before 37 weeks' gestation and in truth the condition is still not well understood with most early births still happening without any clear reason.

The very early signs of labour include: any type of contraction-like sensation; low, dull backache; pelvic pressure or pain; diarrhoea; vaginal spotting; bleeding; and watery vaginal discharge.

If your partner has so much as a scintilla of doubt about something she is feeling, get in touch with your doctor or midwife asap.

67

Assume the position

After the end of this seventh month your baby can no longer turn a somersault in the womb.

That's it, no more fooling around now for the little one; it's time to get ready for the serious stuff.

By the end of this month he or she will measure around 28cm from crown to rump and weigh in at about 3½lbs, which is starting to sound a bit more like a baby's weight isn't it?

As well as fattening up, your baby is continuing to mature and become more independent, ready for going it alone in a few weeks time. He can now control his own body temperature and his bone marrow has now taken complete responsibility for the making of red blood cells.

68

Dodgy pint

Your baby is now passing urine into the amniotic fluid at the rate of about a pint every single day, which is a lot of wee for someone so wee.

Mind you, now they have fully functioning taste buds on their tongue and inside their cheeks they must surely be starting to realise that the amniotic marketing board may have been overegging its product's appeal slightly.

69

May contain nuts

Your baby's brain is starting a growth spurt this month and to squeeze inside its skull it starts to fold over on itself.

This explains why all of our brains take on that weird walnut look.

70

Never refuse a sit down

If you thought your partner was tired in the early weeks of pregnancy, brace yourself for the run in.

Deep-down fatigue will return like an old, crotchety, short-tempered companion that will never really leave either of you for the next two decades.

Enjoy.

71

Clunk click

If you've not done so already, getting hold of a pregnancy seatbelt extension is a very good idea.

It essentially means that in the event of an accident, the belt doesn't put pressure on the bump.

If you buy it unprompted, it also means you are a sensitive, thoughtful and resourceful god among men.

All for a seatbelt.

72

Stroll on

Walking is your friend.

It's not only a great way to spend some time together and talk about how you are both feeling, it also means your partner is getting some gentle but invaluable exercise and fresh air.

73

Give some back up

Back pain is a nightmare at the best of times.

Suffering from it when you're pregnant though is as annoying as it is inevitable. That doesn't mean you can't do something to keep your partner's discomfort to a minimum though.

Buying her a pair of low-heeled or flat shoes that don't look like they have been stolen from a bowling alley is a good start. Gently encouraging her to sit with a straight back on a hard chair or the floor is smart too, although be prepared to be told occasionally to stop acting like her mother.

There are also bump support belts available, which take some of the strain off the back. If you get one of these, under no circumstances refer to it as her truss.

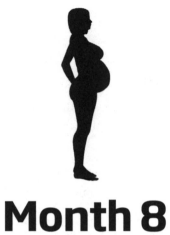

Month 8

74

What's the plan?

A birth plan is a written record intended to be read by the midwives on duty when you go into hospital, of how your partner would like her labour to play out.

Some people structure them chronologically: early stages, transition, delivery etc; others write theirs issue by issue: pain relief, favoured positions, feeding the baby.

As for whether you need one or not, the very act of thinking about and writing the birth plan together as a couple means that you both focus on the potential issues that may arise at a time when you can think clearly and at least go some way to addressing them mentally.

For that reason alone it's got to be a list worth making.

75

Baby you can drive my car

Driving your pregnant partner to the hospital is one of the traditional, cast-iron father-to-be jobs of all time and planning the route is a rite of passage in more ways than one.

If you've not been to a hospital for a few years allow me to also tell you about a major change you may not be familiar with – the revenue generated by hospital car parks now makes up just under 75% of the entire gross national product of the UK.

Or at least that's what it feels like.

Take change, take cash, take gold. If you're in for a long labour you'll need all of them in vast quantities.

76

Not for me, thanks

This is very easily overlooked, but from now on you may be called upon to drive your contracting other half to hospital at any point, so watch your alcohol intake.

With your partner having almost certainly chauffeured you around for the past eight months, it wouldn't look great if you had to drop out of your big behind-the-wheel moment because you'd had a mouthful too much Merlot.

You'll have more than enough on your plate during that journey without hoping beyond hope that a traffic copper doesn't pull you over and take you off the road there and then.

77

Nest is best

Nesting is a very real phenomenon and while it doesn't show itself in all pregnant women it can bring about some pretty frenzied activity.

The hormone prolactin is to blame with tests on animals showing that nesting and nurturing behaviours in both males and females increase the more prolactin is present.

There is though something incredibly humbling about being around a nesting woman.

Nesting essentially brings us down from our self-constructed plinth as a super species and acts as yet another reminder, should we need one, that we are really just monkeys with hats on. I say we, because the urge to nest towards the end of pregnancy doesn't just affect women; you can get caught up in the hormonal house cleaning too – you clucky old thing, you.

78

Stop! Carry on

Choosing when to stop work towards the end of the pregnancy can be a very tricky decision for your partner.

Some women, imagining that they will want to work until the very last second, find themselves dragging their weary bones on public transport and up office stairs wishing that they hadn't been quite so gung-ho early on.

Others, who are lucky enough to have been able to give themselves plenty of time off ahead of the big day, can find themselves bored and marooned at home with hour after hour to think about what awaits them on the big day.

It's a hard one to judge and your role, dear father, is to support and ease her physical and, if needs be, mental woes as much as you can as she enters the final furlongs.

I wouldn't use the furlong analogy mind you.

79

Head down

By the end of this month the average baby weighs in at around 5¼lbs and is a touch over 18 inches long crown to rump.

His main preoccupation at the moment is trying to get himself settled into a head-down position and adjust to the increasing lack of space in the hitherto roomy womb.

Once they have found the slot, as it were, some babies do decide to turn back round again, although attempted escape at this stage is futile.

80

The hard yards

The level of all-round discomfort felt by your partner increases this month on a lot of fronts.

Thanks to a pregnancy hormone called (of course) relaxin, your partner's pelvic joints loosen, expand and therefore unsurprisingly ache in preparation for birth.

There's also more discomfort to be had as the ever-expanding baby forces the womb against your partner's lower ribs as well as the abdomen, which often becomes so stretched that her navel sticks outwards instead of inwards.

She may also notice that her feet and ankles are pretty swollen by the end of the day too thanks to water retention. Perversely, drinking water actually reduces water retention so keep the fluid flowing.

81

Carpal tunnel syndrome

Carpal tunnel syndrome (CTS) is a medical condition in which a nerve in the wrist is compressed, leading to numbness, muscle weakness and pain in the hand.

Symptoms are often worse at night and guess what – pregnant women are highly susceptible to it as weight gain and swelling are also contributory factors. Although not all pregnant women suffer from it, it's estimated that between 20% and 60% do, which is a hell of a lot considering the relatively low profile the condition still has.

Flexing wrists and fingers regularly throughout the day is said to help by some and make matters worse by others, so wrist splints worn at night are often the only treatment of any worth. These keep wrists in a position that provides space in the offending area and eases the problem.

82

Ring the changes

Haemorrhoids, an ugly-looking word for an ugly complaint.

If your partner is suffering on the pile front, buy in a job lot of witch hazel – which is a good natural remedy – and offer to apply it regularly.

It's the very least you can do.

83

Footloose

You've really not got long until you are parents now.

Not long at all.

If your partner can handle it, make the most of your last few weeks of no-babysitter-required freedom. Eat out, go to the cinema, see friends, and lie in; but not necessarily in that order.

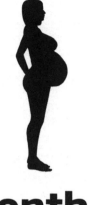

Month 9

84

Not so fast

Welcome to the final month.

Or is it?

Only a miserly 5% of babies arrive bang on the money and out of the remaining 95%, seven in 10 arrive late.

So the odds are that your partner has still got a fair bit of incubating to do yet.

85

Sleep and rest

The most important thing for your partner to do at this stage is to sleep and rest.

The most difficult thing for your partner to do at this stage is to sleep and rest.

86

Nothing to see here

Get into the habit early of politely telling friends and family that you'll let them know as soon as something happens, rather than them needing to ask.

It's a long enough month without having to field daily requests for 'any news' and although reading this you may think me a miserable bastard and that you will never react to people's interest with anything other than unbridled gratitude – I promise eventually it will annoy you to the very core of your being.

87

Cook up a storm

When your baby arrives home you'll be all over the place for a few weeks as the normalities of everyday life, such as eating and sleeping, get hijacked by the new person in the nappy.

While you can't really prepare for the sleep deprivation, you can make moves to ensure you and your bruised and battered partner aren't reduced to consoling yourselves that the corn on the cob in the KFC bucket you've just bought at least constitutes one of your five a day.

Fill the freezer with shepherd's pies, lasagnes, (mild) chillies – whatever nutritious comfort foods you fancy in fact, and you'll be glad to call on this scrumptious stockpile when times get tough.

88

Chill

It sounds obvious, but the pair of you should do your best to relax as much as possible this month.

Walking remains a great option if your partner's up for it and the movement is even thought to bring on labour. Or if something less strenuous is in order go to the pictures or join a postal DVD club and make every night movie night – no birth DVDs though, eh?

As far as you're concerned you could squeeze a last game of golf in – not last game forever, but last for a while – or go to a match. Or – my personal recommendation is stay in bed as much as you can and savour the knowledge that you could get up if you wanted to – but crucially you don't have to.

89

Baby, I'm ready to go

The final pieces of the baby's anatomical jigsaw are put into place this month: the central nervous system is all but fully wired, the digestive system is complete and his lungs mature to full capacity leaving him ready to breathe his first ever breath.

His skin is as smooth and soft as a baby's bottom, especially his bottom, and there is still the odd dollop of the cream-cheese substitute vernix around to help the passage down the birth canal.

He is ready to rock and roll.

90

Coiled spring

Just in case you've forgotten, your partner could go into labour at any second so keep your mobile on, the car full of petrol and your bloodstream free of too much alcohol so you can drive the thing.

And relax.

91

Are we nearly there yet?

For many years, it was believed that the mother's body was responsible for starting labour, but research now points to the baby himself as the one to kick the whole thing off by pressing the hormonal eject button and sending a message to his mum to get a move on.

One theory is that the baby's lungs secrete an enzyme when they are fully developed which triggers contractions; another is that glands near the baby's kidneys do the deed and expel a hormone that starts things moving.

Whatever starts it, one of the most curious things about childbirth is that for something so profound, so dramatically life-changing, it almost always starts with more of a whimper than a bang.

But it soon gets going . . .

92

Labour of love

There are three clear stages of labour:

The first stage is when the neck of the uterus is gradually opened by contractions. This process itself consists of three stages, early labour, active labour and the transitional phase. It's safe to say that these three get progressively more painful.

The second stage is when your partner pushes a new life out into the world.

The third stage is the delivery of the now-redundant placenta.

Prepare to be in awe.

93

And breathe

While you are both at home in the early stages, try to encourage your partner to stay as relaxed and rested as she possibly can, given that every few minutes she is laid low with an ever-increasing pain.

She could watch a favourite film, take a warm (but not hot) bath or just try her best to put her feet up in between the contractions. If she feels hungry, eating and drinking something she fancies is a brilliant move to gain some fuel for the heavy, heavy going ahead.

When she's having a contraction, help her to get in whatever position gives her the most relief. Now's also the time to start using any breathing or relaxation techniques you've learnt at your antenatal classes.

94

Am I nearly 10 yet?

When you arrive at hospital it would be lovely to say that you will be greeted at the door by the midwife who has coached, cared and caressed your partner for the past nine months, but, especially if you live in a city, the chances are that you won't know her.

Whoever it is though will almost certainly go through the same procedure: lots of tests which will culminate in an internal examination to find out how dilated your partner is.

This can be a crushing moment if your partner has been really suffering contraction-wise and feels like she must be a fair way down the road to the magic 10cm, only to find out that she is only 1–2cm gone.

So be prepared to be there for her and tell her how fantastically she is doing.

95

It's a gas

Otherwise known as Entonox, this colourless and odourless gas comprises of half oxygen and half nitrous oxide – or laughing gas. It has the effect of dampening the pain, relaxing the muscles and making the mum-to-be feel a little light-headed; sometimes, just sometimes, even making her laugh.

Gas and air is most often used at the end of the first stage of labour as contractions intensify in frequency and strength. Some women swear by the stuff, but for others it just isn't strong enough, or the light-headedness or even nausea that it can cause puts them off.

It's definitely worth sneaking a quick slug of it yourself if you find a discreet and opportune moment – but don't have too much for Christ's sake.

96

Pethidine

Pethidine is a proper painkiller: part of the opiate family and a synthetic version of morphine.

Administered via injection during the first stage of labour it will help your partner relax and dull the pain by essentially making her as high as a kite.

Sounds great. I'll have some right away please.

Whoa there! Pethidine has its issues, the main one being that it crosses the placenta and can trouble your baby's breathing and make him drowsy for several days, potentially also stifling the baby's rooting and sucking reflexes in the days after birth – making breastfeeding more difficult.

With these issues in mind, if the midwife thinks the baby is just an hour or two away from making an appearance then the pethidine will stay on the drugs trolley.

97

Epidural

The Johnny big bananas of all labour pain relief, an epidural sees painkilling drugs passed into the small of the back via a fine tube.

Official figures show that the numbers of mothers-to-be who have had an epidural has risen in recent years to a whopping 36.5% of all births in the UK.

The pros and cons of the procedure are debated endlessly, but can be crudely summed up thus in terms of your partner's choices – complete pain relief versus complete birth experience.

98

Hoover or tongs?

Things don't always go to plan of course during labour.

Your baby might be getting distressed or your partner simply might have zero energy left to push. Around one in eight UK births are assisted using instruments. There is the ventouse – a cup with a pulling handle attached to it, which is then linked to a small vacuum pump – being one method.

Sophisticated, it's not.

Then even more rudimentary are forceps – and although these have a higher success rate than ventouse, your partner is also more likely to sustain some damage with their use.

Neither route is pretty, but there comes a point in labour when the baby needs to come out sharpish for its own safety.

99

The sunroof exit

If after three attempts with the forceps your baby is still refusing to move it's almost certainly time to stop tugging and think about a caesarean section.

A Caesarean section (C-section) involves making an incision into the woman's abdomen and uterus to manually remove the baby. A screen is usually put up while it takes place so you and your partner don't have to witness what's going on – many men can't resist a peek though and some regret it given what they then see.

While a c-section is a serious medical procedure, it can be over remarkably quickly and before you know where you are, after hours and hours of labour you can suddenly be holding your new baby.

As you'd expect after having major surgery, your partner will be pretty immobile and in considerable pain for a good while afterwards, meaning your role once you get home becomes even more crucial too.

100

Give me some skin

Immediately after your baby is born, if all is well with both mother and child, skin-to-skin contact will be established between the two without delay to start the bonding process.

There's also plenty of evidence to suggest that you should get your shirt off and get close to your little one too at some point, as well as fixing his gaze with yours – both of which are thought to help form a lasting bond between you and your new child.

One job that needs to be done before you do that is the cutting of the umbilical cord. The midwife will clamp it in two places and if you wish you can do the honours in what has become a well-practised symbolic gesture of the establishing of true independence.

In reality it's like cutting a very tough and gristly German sausage.

101

You're the daddy!

Your first experience of childbirth will never leave you. Shocking or sentimental, traumatic or transformational – the memories of the moment you became a father and what your partner went through to make that happen will live as long as you do.

No matter what friends who've been there tell you ahead of the event, no matter what you see on the television or at the movies and no matter what you read, yes even in books like this one, nothing even gets close to how you will feel.

Cherish every moment of this day and the days that follow it as you burst with pride for your new family – it really is life at its very best.

Need more tips and advice?
Get the full version of Pregnancy for Men

"Made me laugh out loud and pretty useful too"
Pregnancy & birth magazine

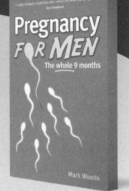

Most pregnancy books are for women but this is a highly humorous survival guide for fathers, guiding them through nine months of joy, excitement and fear, including:

✓ Advice on how to support the pregnant mum

✓ Month-by-month updates on your baby's growth and development

✓ Stories and tips from other expectant dads

amazon.co.uk

Available on Amazon.co.uk

amazonkindle

Also available as an ebook on Amazon Kindle

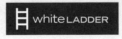

www.whiteladderpress.co.uk

Get 101 tips to prepare you for fatherhood...

Includes enlightening and funny quotes from new dads

Now you've successfully navigated the maze of pregnancy, what happens when your bundle of joy finally arrives? Mark Woods is on hand to give you 101 witty and insightful tips to help you become the best dad in town, including:

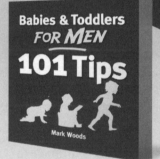

✓ Essential man-to-man advice
✓ Advice on how to support mum
✓ Changing nappies, potty training and much more

amazon.co.uk
Available on Amazon.co.uk

amazonkindle
Also available as an ebook on Amazon Kindle

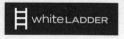

www.whiteladderpress.co.uk